Why I Don't Jog, Play Tennis, Bicycle, Swim, Row or Dance

Published by:
Quinlan Press
131 Beverly Street
Boston, MA 02114

Cover illustration and design by Edgar Stewart

Library of Congress Cataloging-in-Publication Data

McCann, Thomas P.
Why I don't jog, play tennis, bicycle, swim, row, or dance.

Bibliography: p.
1. Heart—Diseases—Mortality. 2. Sudden death.
3. Obituaries. 4. Exercise—Physiological effect.
I. Siegel, Arthur J. II. Title.
RC682.M38 1987 616.1'2078 87-43042
ISBN 0-933341-06-7

Why I Don't Jog, Play Tennis, Bicycle, Swim, Row or Dance

by
Thomas P. McCann

with a medical perspective
provided by
Arthur J. Siegel, M.D.
Medical Director, Hahnemann Hospital
Assistant Clinical Professor of Medicine,
Harvard Medical School

QUINLAN PRESS
Boston

This one's for Jackie Gleason, "The Great One," who broke all the rules, lived long enough and enjoyed every minute.

Why I Wrote This Book

For as long as I can remember, I've believed in the ''number's up'' theory. Simply stated, it means that when your number's up, it's up, and you die. It doesn't matter whether you're two, twenty-two, or a hundred and two. Nor does it matter who you are, what you do, or what you have done. It doesn't even matter what ''shape'' you are in.

That's what this book is all about.

I wrote—or ''assembled'' would be more appropriate—this book for a very good purpose and for a large audience of much maligned and demeaned readers. It's for the person who refuses to exercise, no matter what. If you are one of these people, your reasons are your business; the important thing is to shuck off the guilt trip foisted on you by the fitness and vitality clique. With this book you've got the ammunition to debunk the well promoted myth that heavy exercise is good for your health or will prolong your life. What's more, you've got a lot of good examples with which to needle your so-called ''in shape'' friends.

About twenty years ago I began to notice a self-styled elite emerging which was equally convinced that the "number's up" theory was wrong—and they alone possessed the secret to staying the chilly tap of the Guy who calls out the numbers. The members of this cult make a commitment to health and fitness at various ages; sometimes they make it early and stay with it for life, sometimes in middle age, sometimes in old age. They take their vows before an altar bedecked with offerings of yogurt, raw vegetables, brie and designer water with slices of lime. Until recently I thought they threw in the lime for nourishment, but one of "them" (actually, my daughter Nancy, a jogger) told me they use it for its diuretic properties, to help them expell the dollar-a-pint water.

Many break their vows and fall off the fitness wagon, but a great many of them stay with it for life—if you can call it a life. The fact is, after a lifetime of relentless jogging, swimming, tennis, squash, golf, preaching and plotting, death usually occurs in their group at about the three-score and ten mark (that's seventy for those of you younger readers who don't know what "score" means in the numerical sense). Funny thing is, this is exactly where death usually occurs in my group. One recent example is Jackie Gleason who broke all the rules—drank too much, smoked four packs a day, ate anything and everything in sight, was always at least a hundred pounds overweight, never broke a sweat—and died on the dot of three score and ten. So being in or out of shape really doesn't matter.

I am always amazed when people who dedicate their lives to strenuous exercise live as long as they do considering they have never learned to relax. I'll give them one thing, however; they do make the best-looking corpses.

These health, fitness and vitality freaks, whose hidden agenda is to dump guilt on the less active among us, first came to the world's attention in 490 B.C. (Before Calories, that is). It seems that one spring day that year, a Greek courier scampered more than twenty-six miles to bring news of a key victory over the Persians. Today, Persians are known as Iranians and are doing much better since they changed their name. Unfortunately, for this early roadrunner, legend has it that he forgot to "cool down" and dropped dead on the spot.

The Greeks hailed the victory of course, but got really excited and hailed the runners feat (not to be confused with the runners feet which, legend has it, were generally scorned) in the *Papyrus Daily Press*. The publicity gave birth to the famed marathon, which is contested annually and most notably in my adopted Boston. Today marathons all over the world provide an excellent excuse for millions of exhibitionists to expose themselves clad only in jock straps and flimsy shorts to millions of voyeurs.

I must admit that until the age of about thirty-five I too performed certain bodily maneuvers, usually with inflated leather balls, which helped classify me as being "in shape." I must also admit that until age thirty-five I was an officer of a Fortune

500 company and thus was always in a nervous, unhappy, worried state which helped keep me thin, pale and pained-looking, so people assumed I was healthy and in shape. Happily, I had the intelligence to quit the job and slip into a life of lethargy, writing and producing television shows.

Simultaneously, my shift from the active to the sedentary life served to heighten my unusual, albeit somewhat morbid, hobby of collecting the obituaries of people who died while exercising. Each of these documented deaths, which quickly filled a fat file, only reassured me in a perverse way that I had found the key to a long and healthy life. Friends began to send me obits to add to my collection. At last, I had tangible proof of something I had always suspected: the joy of movement movement is not all it's cracked up to be.

Imagine my sense of well-being while reading the obituaries of such exercise victims as the guru of the U.S. jogging craze who died in the act, or the 38-year-old artist who suffered a fatal heart attack while exercising at an American Heart Association fundraiser. And how about the macho film star who dropped dead while jogging along an Irish country road? And then there's the racquetball champion who collapsed and died, also at 38, while playing racquetball.

Exercise can be hazardous to your health in other ways; for example, the out-of-town businessman who was shot dead in New Orleans while jogging, not to mention the reports of the scores of joggers attacked by birds and run over by cars, trucks, motorcycles, even skateboarders. How about the U.S. senator who died after performing a song-and-dance routine at a Press Club benefit? The list is long. Very long. Each new obituary lets me rest more easily—while still breathing, of course. In fact, exercise can be so lethal that I have written to the Surgeon General to suggest he look into exercise products with a view toward labeling them "Dangerous To Your Health."

I woke up one day to the realization that I had become an amateur necrologist. My interest compels me each day to turn first to the obituary page (which some refer to as "the Irish sports page"). I just have to know what people did with their lives and what did them in. I began to try my hand at rewriting a few obits I thought could have been improved upon, or contained errors, or ones I thought were given short shrift by the obit writer.

In time, friends who knew of my interest and newly acquired ability to write superb obituaries began to ask me to write theirs. Some wanted them written even before they died. One good friend just three weeks before his death called me to his bedside and asked me to write his obit. He summed it up: "Why should I permit some undertaker or a stranger on a newspaper to botch up my life and run the risk of him leaving out something important when there's somebody like you, Tom, ready, willing and, let's face it, eager to write it for me?" Of course I did it for him and he died content.

In recent years I have also had the pleasure of writing my own obituary carefully detailing a host of wonderful accomplishments. I keep it in my top drawer, and everyone knows it's there. It is a very thoughtful thing to have done for my wife Joan, and our children, Alison, Lynn, Nancy and Peter. God knows I've done enough obituaries in my lifetime to know what a scramble there always is to assemble the facts, organize them and compile a list of publications to send it to, etc. It's a real chore, and if a member of the family has to do it, it's just an additional bit of needless grief. But it's got to be done, someone's got to do it, and it's important—at least to me.

So, in the interest of saving someone a lot of trouble (and also in the interest of getting the facts straight), I have done it myself. I have even specified the distribution list, short but complete, consisting of the *Boston Globe,* the *New York Times, Variety,* the *Boston Herald* and *New York News* (for my friends who only read tabloids) and the *Bulletin of the Algonquin Club of Boston.* I have told all the family members that I want the coolest one among them to follow my detailed instructions. All he or she will have to do is fill in a couple of blanks, i.e., the when, where and how parts. I update the text and photo annually, which is a lot more than I do with regard to the condition of my health. I feel really good about it and secure in the knowledge that none of my good deeds in life will be omitted and none of my bad deeds included. I even dream about seeing it in print.

Like Mark Twain, I wish at times that I too could observe that "the reports of my death are greatly exaggerated." It would be exciting to read one's printed obituary while still alive. My real fantasy is to see my own unedited version printed in the *New York Sunday Times,* complete with the photo taken by my professional photographer daughter Lynn. (How much more meaningful, even poetic, it would be to have her credit on my obit photo than to have Fabian Bachrach's credit. And how good the exposure would be for her business.)

None of us knows when or how we're going to die, and that's good. It's hard enough for most human beings to live with the knowledge that someday they *will.* If we knew when, where, how. . . that would be too much. One of the great comedians, now dead—it might have been Durante, Groucho, W.C. Fields or none of the above—once said that if he knew where he was going to die he "wouldn't be caught dead there." I always liked that line, but then again, I would. In that same vein and spirit, one thing I'm absolutely sure about is that I'll never be caught dead jogging, playing tennis or golf, swimming, rowing, bicycling or anything remotely resembling heavy physical activity. When I die, I want people to know I've been sick.

Tom McCann
Boston
August, 1987

[redacted], 49

[redacted] physician

[redacted], 49, a [redacted] physician, died on Thursday afte having a heart seizure while play ing basketball.

Dr. [redacted] had a private practice in [redacted] for the past [redacted] years and was also a membe of the staff at [redacted].

[redacted].

[redacted]

[redacted], a former [redacted], died Tuesday. He had suffered a heart attack while playing golf in [redacted] He was 79 years old and lived in [redacted].

[redacted]

[redacted]

[redacted] of [redacted].

[redacted], 53, Dies; Designed a [redacted]

[redacted], professor of [redacted] science at the [redacted], died of a heart attack while jogging on the campus of Johns Hopkins University in Baltimore. He was 53 years old and lived in [redacted]

Professor [redacted] was doing research at [redacted]; he was on a leave of absence from [redacted]

[redacted]

Memorial service at [redacted] for [redacted], 53

A memorial service will be held at [redacted] of [redacted]

Dr. [redacted] and a friend were fly fishing [redacted] on the [redacted] in [redacted], when [redacted] was suddenly swept away by rushing water that was released by a dam upstream, according to [redacted], [redacted]

[redacted], 38, racquetball exec

[redacted] the 38-year-old chairman of the [redacted] collapsed and died while playing racquetball.

[redacted] a resident of [redacted] collapsed Thursday at [redacted] Racquet Club in [redacted] where he had gone on Racquetball Association business. He died shortly afterward at [redacted] Hospital.

[redacted]

OBITUARIES

[redacted], 76; former [redacted],

[redacted]

[redacted] died here yesterday after suffering a heart attack while playing golf at the [redacted] Golf Club.

Mr. [redacted] was pronounced dead at [redacted] Hospital. He was 76.

[redacted]

In [redacted]

[redacted] Olympic leader, [redacted], while jogging; in-law dies hours later

[redacted]

[redacted] – [redacted] Olympic [redacted] medalist and [redacted] died of a heart attack as he jogged Saturday, police said. He was 58.

[redacted] body, clad in running clothes, was found at a [redacted] intersection about 9:30 a.m., said police Lt. [redacted] He said it was not known immediately who it was because Mr. [redacted] wore no identification.

[redacted] who won a bronze medal in the [redacted]."

"I got a lot out of sports, and I'd like to contribute something back," said Mr. [redacted] a lifelong rower, swimmer and amateur sports enthusiast.

Mr. [redacted] also competed in Olymnpic Games in [redacted], [redacted] and [redacted] In [redacted] he won the [redacted] Award as the nation's outstanding amateur athlete.

Hours after Mr. [redacted] death, his brother-in-law died, apparently of a heart attack, while walking, said [redacted]

Dr. [redacted], chief medical examiner for the county [redacted] said in a statement released Saturday evening, "They are apparently unconnected but we have no statement.

'[redacted] was found dead at about 9:30 this morning in a jogging outfit. His brother-in-law was found dead in street clothes at about 4:30 p.m. We are hoping, but are not yet ready to state, it is a coincidence."

[redacted], 66, host of television's "[redacted]"

[redacted]

[redacted] – Television [redacted] producer and star [redacted] died yesterday while jogging in Central Park, hospital officials said. He was 66.

Mr. [redacted] who created the popular daytime [redacted] show "T[redacted]" and hosted it for the [redacted]s, was pronounced dead at [redacted]l about 1:20 p.m., a hospital spokeswoman said. The exact cause of death was not immediately released.

Mr. [redacted] was jogging in Manhattan's Central Park near 64th street and Fifth avenue when he collapsed, a hospital spokeswoman said.

[redacted]."

[redacted]

[redacted], 49, partner in [redacted]y died [redacted] of an apparent heart attack while playing softball in [redacted]f. [redacted] Softball Competition Benefit when he was stricken. He was pronounced dead on arrival at [redacted]t Hospital.

[redacted], [redacted] at [redacted]

[redacted] 51

[redacted]

Funeral services will be held at [redacted] in the [redacted] in North Easton for [redacted], [redacted]l.

[redacted], of [redacted] who [redacted], died unexpectedly Friday while playing golf in the [redacted] Tournament at the [redacted] Golf Course in [redacted] He was 51.

[redacted]

[redacted], died last night about two hours after apparently suffering a heart attack while pitching batting practice for the [redacted] He was 57.

Mr. [redacted] had been working for the [redacted] as an instructional coach and scout and threw batting practice prior to almost every [redacted] home game.

Joggers' latest problem: bird attacks

[redacted]

Forget frost bite, heat stroke and muscle strain. European doctors have documented an even more stinging hazard of jogging: bird attacks.

Over the last two years, physicians at Kantonsspital Liestal in Liestal, Switzerland, say they have cared for 12 joggers who were attacked by birds.

"The birds attacked by diving from behind and continuing to dive as long as joggers were in motion," wrote Dr. P. Itin and colleagues in today's New England Journal of Medicine.

Five joggers identified the birds as European buzzards.

The victims, all men attacked between April and July, suffered head cuts up to six inches long.

[redacted]

after $3\frac{1}{8}$-mile [redacted] race; at 29

Dr. [redacted] 29, of [redacted] a major in the [redacted] was buried with a 21-gun military salute Saturday in [redacted] Cemetery in [redacted]. A memorial service had been held earlier in the [redacted]

[redacted] was competing in an interservice decathlon event with [redacted] at the Olympic Stadium in Munich, Germany, on [redacted] when he collapsed after a 5000-meter ($3\frac{1}{8}$ miles) race. He died the following day, the same day that he was promoted to [redacted]

[redacted]

[redacted] man, 58, dies while jogging

A 58-year-old [redacted] man collapsed and died yesterday morning while jogging around [redacted], according to [redacted] Police. [redacted] of [redacted] avenue was pronounced dead at [redacted] Hospital after apparently suffering a heart attack, a spokeswoman said.

Family members said Mr. [redacted] a [redacted] who was active in [redacted] community affairs, was a regular jogger and swimmer.

Mr. [redacted] was found lying unconscious near the asphalt path used by joggers at [redacted] at 6:45 a.m. by [redacted], police said. [redacted] said he recognized [redacted] from numerous other morning runs along the pond.

[redacted] said he ran across the street to his home to call an ambulance. He said his wife, [redacted] a nurse at [redacted], performed mouth-to-mouth resuscitation on [redacted] while waiting for emergency help.

[redacted] Coach

[redacted]

[redacted] the head football coach at [redacted] University, died of an apparent heart attack Saturday morning while jogging in [redacted], where he was vacationing with his family. He was 44 years old.

[redacted]

[redacted] Jr., 68, *Ex-Editor of* [redacted]

[redacted] former executive editor of [redacted] and [redacted] magazines, died Friday after being stricken by a heart attack while running in [redacted] State Forest. He was 68 years old and lived on [redacted] and in [redacted].

A lifelong journalist, Mr. [redacted] accompanied United States troops during the liberation of Europe and later led [redacted] for six years.

He graduated from [redacted] in [redacted] and joined the [redacted], [redacted]

[redacted] Dead at 51; Member of [redacted]

[redacted]

Former Representative [redacted], a member of the House [redacted] Committee during the [redacted], died Thursday night in [redacted]. He turned 51 years old Thursday and lived in [redacted].

[redacted] who represented [redacted] from 1968 until 1976, apparently suffered a heart attack while playing tennis. He was taken to [redacted], where he died at 6 P.M.

[redacted]’’

“[redacted] his [redacted].

[redacted], “[redacted] of [redacted]

[redacted]

[redacted]

[redacted]

[redacted] DIES JOGGING

[redacted]

WRITER [redacted] 52, whose best-selling books [redacted] collapsed and died from a heart attack while running down a country road in northern [redacted] his family said yesterday.

[redacted], was wearing jogging shorts and running shoes when his body was found on Route [redacted].

A passing motorcyclist spotted the [redacted] body at about 5 p.m. Friday, 100 yards from the [redacted] where he had checked in just an hour before.

[redacted]

According to [redacted] who performed an autopsy yesterday, [redacted] "had serious heart disease affecting two major arteries to the heart. They were completely blocked off.

"He never had any warning. If he did, he ignored it,"

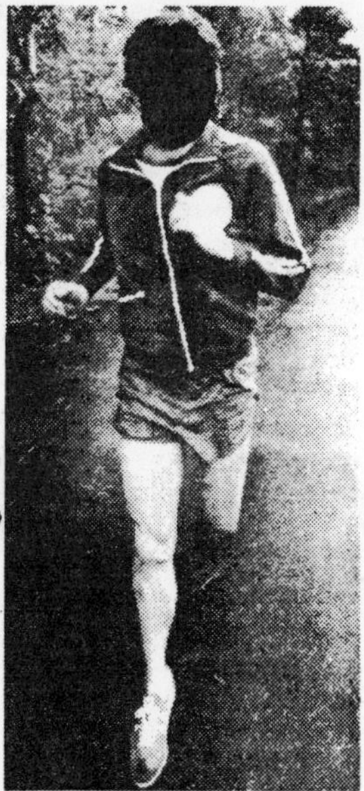

[redacted] . . . [redacted]

said [redacted] chief medical examiner.

Except for his heart, she

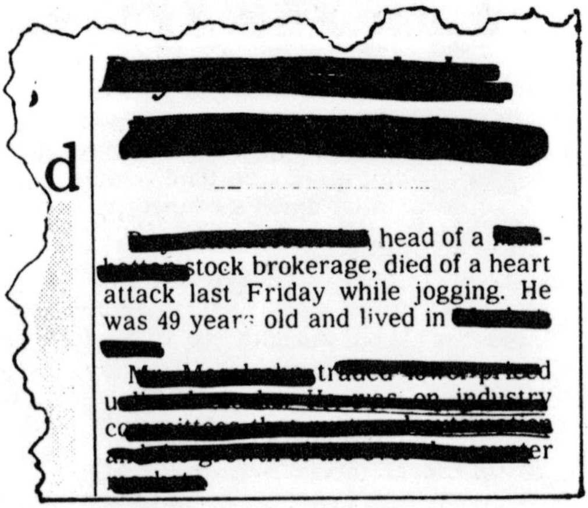

d

[redacted]

[redacted], head of a [redacted]-[redacted] stock brokerage, died of a heart attack last Friday while jogging. He was 49 years old and lived in [redacted].

[redacted] tr[redacted]d u[redacted] c[redacted]er [redacted]

[redacted] 52

Sales representative

[redacted] – A funeral Mass will be said today at 10 a.m. in [redacted]'s Church, [redacted], for [redacted], 52, of [redacted] a sales representative in [redacted] for the [redacted] a manufacturer of [redacted]. [redacted] died after suffering a heart attack while playing handball during a business trip to [redacted] on Thursday. He was pronounced dead in the [redacted].

[redacted]

[redacted] man, 61, shot to death while jogging in [redacted]

[redacted] – A [redacted] businessman was shot and killed while jogging, when he refused to stop for a robber in a tough downtown neighborhood. A 17-year-old was later booked on a charge of first-degree murder.

[redacted], of [redacted]., was shot once in the back of the head when he refused to stop for a man who ran up behind him, witnesses told police after the Saturday shooting. The gunman took a gold bracelet and fled, police said.

Officers said [redacted] had set out jogging from his [redacted] hotel and apparently was not aware that he headed near the La- [redacted]

A few blocks past the project, the man ran up behind him and began talking, but [redacted] did not stop, witnesses said.

[redacted]

for-
arch
hus-
an).
aren,
Son
rman
[redacted]
ohn,
Eliz-
re
m.
d.
at
st,
arly
and
oted
of
en-
vin
via
d

OBITUARIES

[redacted], 54

Vice president of [redacted] firm

[redacted]., 54, of [redacted] died Sunday in [redacted] after apparently suffering a heart attack while on a skiing vacation with his family in the [redacted] area.

[redacted]er b[redacted]o.

[redacted] a[redacted].

OBITUARIES

[redacted], 52

[redacted]

[redacted] – [redacted], 52, of [redacted] a retired [redacted] in the [redacted] State Police, died Sunday while jogging. He apparently suffered a heart attack and was pronounced dead at [redacted].

[redacted]

[redacted]

[redacted]

[redacted]

[redacted], Calif., Feb. 7 [redacted] — [redacted], whose [redacted] renditions of [redacted] appeared in [redacted] for nearly a decade, died of a heart attack Saturday after exercising at a fund-raiser for the American Heart Association. He was 38 years old.

The artist, one of about 25 celebrities who worked out for about 15 minutes as part of [redacted]

[redacted]

[redacted]

[redacted] 32

Worked with [redacted]

[redacted], 32, of [redacted] a [redacted] worker and program coordinator, died unexpectedly Thursday while playing basketball.

Born in [redacted] attended the [redacted]

[redacted] 58

[redacted]

[redacted] 58, [redacted], died Saturday from injuries sustained in a skiing accident in Aspen.

[redacted]

[redacted] Death By Heat Stroke Is Investigated

[redacted]

[redacted] — The State Health Department is investigating the actions of a [redacted] hospital where a city official died of heat stroke after running in a 10-kilometer road race [redacted].

The official, [redacted], [redacted], remained unconscious in the emergency department of the hospital, [redacted] Hospital, for more than two hours without his temperature having been taken and without any effort having been made to cool him down, according to [redacted], [redacted], who reported the case to the state Wednesday.

The hospital staff began treating Mr. [redacted], 34 years old, for heat stroke when he entered the intensive care unit, [redacted] said. By that time, his temperature was 106.7 degrees and he was suffering seizures, he added.

Stricken hiker dies in mountains

[redacted] – [redacted], 56, of [redacted]., died while hiking on [redacted], apparently the victim of a heart attack, police said, was in a party of four when he was stricken Saturday night on 5,715-foot [redacted] [redacted]. State Police said rescue crews did not reach him until yesterday. (AP)

[redacted]

[redacted]

[redacted], died of a heart attack Saturday while playing in a squash tournament in [redacted] He was 65 years old.

[redacted]

Bo King Y., M Chil

[redacted]

[redacted], a former international banking executive, died of a heart attack Saturday while playing tennis in [redacted], where he lived. He was 62 years old.

[redacted]

[redacted]

[redacted] *Is Dead;*
[redacted] *Announcer*

[redacted] a television announcer for [redacted] who had been the original radio commentator for the [redacted], died yesterday after apparently suffering a heart attack while jogging at a [redacted] health club. He was 51 years old. After collapsing on the track, he was taken to [redacted] City Hospital, where he died.

[redacted]

[redacted]

[redacted], dead at 58

[redacted] — [redacted] who died of a heart attack soon after performing in an [redacted] benefit.

Mr. [redacted] 58, who had a history of heart trouble, was stricken late Friday after singing and dancing in the [redacted] annual fund-raising show, a musical revue that pokes fun at current events.

[redacted]

[redacted]57,
[redacted]
Killed in a Collision

[redacted] was killed Wednesday in Manhattan in an accident while riding her bicycle. She was 57 years old.

The [redacted] died instantly when her bicycle collided with a tractor-trailer on [redacted]

[redacted]

[redacted] 44, Is Dead; Former [redacted] Tennis Star

[redacted], one of [redacted] most successful tennis players in the [redacted] collapsed and died of a heart attack Tuesday while playing golf. He was 44 years old.

[redacted]

Fleet eases older sailors' fitness test

[redacted]

[redacted] – The commander of the [redacted] Fleet, concerned about a colleague who suffered a fatal heart attack while running, has eased a fitness test for sailors under his command who are 45 and older.

The change affects only the [redacted] Fleet but officials at the [redacted] Fleet said they plan to reconsider the Navy fitness regulations.

Adm. [redacted] told the [redacted] Fleet last week that servicemen 45 and older who were once required to complete a 1½-mile run to be considered physically fit must instead finish a 3-mile timed walk.

"The Navy can ill afford to lose more personnel to unnecessary heart attacks," [redacted] told his command. "I expect you to be physically fit. I don't expect you to die getting there."

[redacted]' action was prompted by the [redacted] death of [redacted] Adm. [redacted], 52, commander of the [redacted]e [redacted] collapsed after jogging and died of a heart attack.

There have been a handful of other cases involving senior officers and enlisted members who died after routine jogging. In [redacted], Vice Adm. [redacted], 53, commander of the [redacted]e, collapsed and died while jogging at the Norfolk Naval Air Station in October 1983.

[redacted] 56,

Former [redacted]

[redacted]

[redacted]

[redacted], the director of [redacted], died Saturday after he suffered a heart attack while playing tennis in [redacted] He was 56 years old and lived in [redacted]

[redacted]

was resp ible develop-

[redacted] 43, Dies; Was Criminal Lawyer

[redacted] a criminal defense lawyer in New York City, died Tuesday in [redacted]. The 43-year-old lawyer drowned while swimming in the Atlantic Ocean. He lived in Manhattan.

[redacted].

[redacted] Is Dead at 55; A Former [redacted]

[redacted], a former [redacted], died Monday at [redacted] in [redacted]. He had suffered a heart attack after swimming at the [redacted].

[redacted] was 55 years old and lived in [redacted].

[redacted]

[redacted], 61

Headed [redacted] food firm

[redacted]

[redacted]. – [redacted] president and chief executive officer of [redacted]., the [redacted] company, died Sunday after suffering a heart attack while playing golf. He was 61.

[redacted], a native of [redacted] who joined [redacted] in 1955, was pronounced dead at [redacted] Hospital, said company spokesman [redacted].

[redacted] was appointed chief executive officer in [redacted] and was expected to be named chairman of the [redacted] company at the annual shareholders meeting on [redacted].

John [redacted] 52, air personality on [redacted] since 1971, died Nov. 27 of hardening of arteries-related heart attack while completing scuba diving course at suburban [redacted] swimming pool. He began his broadcasting career at [redacted], and later worked at [redacted]. In addition to his Monday-Saturday [redacted], he also syndicated [redacted] through his own production company, [redacted]

[redacted] 38

Owned a [redacted] business

[redacted] 38, of [redacted], formerly of [redacted] died Monday in [redacted] Hospital, [redacted] of injuries suffered in a bicycle accident in [redacted].

Born in [redacted], [redacted] was graduated from [redacted] at- [redacted].

[redacted] Mr. [redacted]

[redacted]

[redacted]

[redacted] Is Dead at 56; Ran Marathon in Olympics

[redacted]

[redacted], a member of the [redacted] United States Olympic marathon team and a familiar competitor in [redacted] distance and cross-country races, collapsed and died Monday night during a cross-country practice run at [redacted]. He was 56 years old.

Born in [redacted], Mr. [redacted] came to the United States in [redacted]. He became a United States citizen in [redacted] and worked as a [redacted]. He competed for the [redacted] in the 19[redacted], establishing himself as one of the nation's top distance runners.

He finished [redacted] in the marathon in the [redacted] Summer Games in [redacted]. In the [redacted] Pan American Games at [redacted], he won the 10,000 meters and finished third in the marathon.

[redacted], [redacted].

He
les
of
s
h
n-
9
a
be-
ial

[redacted] 52

Assistant principal in [redacted]

[redacted], 52, of [redacted], assistant principal of [redacted] Junior High School, [redacted], died Saturday in [redacted] City Hospital after he suffered a heart attack while jogging in [redacted]

[redacted] died of a heart attack today while working out at a local gymnasium. He was 50 years old.

[redacted]

[redacted] slightly paunchy, a tad jowly and very happy

[redacted]

RIGOROUS AVOIDANCE of physical exercises and the permanent suspension of all dietary controls have left [redacted] exactly where he wants to be at 54 or so — slightly paunchy, a tad jowly and very happy.

[redacted] a dapper gentleman standing 5-foot-7 with a short-clipped mustache, guards his sedentary lifestyle jealously and finances it with the handsome salary he has drawn over the past seven seasons for portraying [redacted] gins on "[redacted]

To top it off, he enjoys his work. Immensely.

Each work day, he escapes physical exertion by taking an elevator from the living room of his 11-room, 38th floor penthouse condominium with a 360-degree view of [redacted] in [redacted] to a waiting chauffeur-driven limousine whisking him off to the [redacted]

Preserving his energy, [redacted] reverses the procedure each evening.

With four months of vacation time to worry about each year, [redacted] recently purchased a second home in the exclusive mountain community of [redacted] a two-hour drive east o[redacted]

The three-level, colonial-style home features 7,000 square feet of living space, six bedrooms and eight bathrooms.

But the compact [redacted] idea of a perfect day is "in bed with a great book and the phones off the hook," smoking two packs of cigarettes through a long holder in the process.

A marvelous evening usually entails renting six video cassettes for marathon viewing of recent films on his big-screen television.

A special evening is usually capped by a gourmet meal and a first class restaurant catering to his special dietary needs, according to [redacted], "which means good food in just the right quantity. I eat anything that appeals to me. I drink. I smoke. I've always been blessed with good health and never been seriously ill. I'm sure someday it will catch up with me, but until then I'm not going to whine about it."

Other than nicer places to live and a measure of financial security, his lifestyle hasn't changed very much over the years.

"I've never been a party animal and I've always been fairly reclusive," says [redacted] "I prefer home to any luxury hotel and have the same small, select group of friends. I don't travel much, but it's nice to know that I could go to London anytime without worrying about paying for the trip."

[redacted] has come a long way since his humble beginning in [redacted], where his father operated a gas station and his mother a beauty parlor.

"To me, doing [redacted] in '[redacted] is the best job I've ever had," [redacted] says. "I could do the character for another 10 years without getting bored."

A Medical Perspective

Exercise and Sudden Cardiac Death: Protection Versus Provocation or How To Reduce the Risk To Reap the Benefit

Arthur J. Siegel, M.D.

It has recently been demonstrated that nonfatal myocardial infarction and sudden death are more likely to occur between 6 a.m. and noon than during other times of the day. New England Journal of Medicine 1987; 316:1514-8.[1]

This recent statistical association of an increase in fatal and nonfatal myocardial events in the morning hours does not necessarily imply that we should remain in bed, although Tom McCann might well choose this option. The dramatic decline in mortality from acute myocardial infarction of the last decade coincides with many changes in the American lifestyle, including the controversial "exercise boom." How do we weigh the putative benefit of regular aerobic exercise accruing to 20 million adult Americans in part from physical activity against the rare, but vexing, occurences of sudden death assembled in his log? While nearly every individual can benefit from a program of regular, moderate physical activity, exercise is not without its hazards. The challenge raised by the assembled obituaries is not to abandon exercise in panic, but to examine critically how to approach exercise to maximize its benefits and reduce its hazards.

Numerous studies have found that regular physical activity protects against morbidity and mortality from coronary heart disease. Paffenbarger's ongoing study of college alumni indicates that the relative risk of death from heart disease is 40 percent lower in individuals who remain physically active through their advancing years in comparison with sedentary classmates. The most recent data from this study justify the following assertion as published by its authors: "By age eighty, the amount of additional life attributable to adequate exercise as compared with sedentariness was one to more than two years."[2]

While there is firm medical and physiologic evidence to indicate that the normal heart benefits from moderate or strenuous physical activity, exercise may provoke problems such as myocardial ischemia, dysrhythmias and even sudden cardiac death in individuals with significant (possibly silent) coronary heart disease. Adequate medical screening and clearance for exercise is imperative, especially in previously sedentary middle-aged men in whom the risk for underlying coronary atherosclerosis may approach one chance in twenty. Risk factors such as hypertension, cigarette smoking and high cholesterol warrant pre-exercise screening tests such as exercise electrocardiography and radionuclide cardioscintigraphy to exclude significant but silent myocardial ischemia with exercise.

The absence of warning signs for heart disease in such screening test constitutes a green light for undertaking a moderate exercise program. The benefits of exercise including walking are real, and even previously sedentary individuals can over several months approach the guidelines approved for aerobic fitness by the American College of Sports Medicine: twenty to thirty minutes of sustained low intensity exercise three to four times per week. The benefits of sustaining physical fitness in this way clearly outweigh the markedly reduced risks which have been eliminated by appropriate screening and medical clearance. The key to safety is consistency over time, and moderate to low exercise intensity.

Some recent studies have demonstrated the overall cardiovascular benefit from regular exercise in direct relationship to sudden cardiac death.[3] The risk for fatal cardiac events decreases in individuals with higher levels of physical activity compared to less active men, although within each activity group the risk of sudden cardiac death during exercise is greater than during sleep or sedentary intervals. Sudden exertion in customarily sedentary individuals presents the absolute highest risk. This builds on prior data from the Framingham study showing that increasing levels of relative inactivity confer a greater cardiac risk.

The prudent recommendation from these data is to build exercise into one's routine on a regular basis but with an emphasis on moderation. Weekend athletic commandos take a high risk of encountering the medical consequences of overexertion including sudden collapse, and extreme levels of exercise such as long distance or marathon running confer higher levels of risk without a proven increment in benefit.

To exercise or not to exercise is not really in question. The issue is how much of a good thing is too much for a given individual, which must take into account one's medical profile, predispositions and lifestyle objectives. Medical guidance and assessment in undertaking an exercise program can minimize the potential hazards so that an individual can safely reap the benefits which exercise physiology and epidemiologic studies have proven exists. The risks of course cannot be reduced to zero, but few things in life are engraved in stone—and we would all like to postpone the ones that are!

Should running shoes be imprinted with a warning that "Exercise May Be Hazardous To Your Health"? McCann seems to argue that the Surgeon General has been off his mark. Abstinence from exercise because of the relatively unusual instances of sudden cardiac death, however, would be akin to abandoning sex because of the AIDS virus threat. Most of us would aspire to a little more than the sedentary and celibate life.[4] "Safe sex" presupposes some degree of whole-body fitness.

REFERENCES

1. Geoffrey H. Tofler, M.B., et al: Concurrent Morning Increase In Platelet Aggregability and the Risk of Myocardial Infarction and Sudden Cardiac Death. (N Engl J Med 1987; 316:1514-8.)

2. Ralph S. Paffenbarger, Jr., M.D., et al: Physical Activity, All-Cause Mortality, and Longevity of College Alumni. (N Engl J Med 1986; 314:605-13.)

3. D. S. Siscovick, et al: The Incidence of Primary Cardiac Arrest During Vigorous Exercise. (N Engl J Med 1984; 311 (Oct 4): 874-7.)

4. St. Augustine, The Confessions Of

Arthur J. Siegel, M.D., *is medical director of the Hahnemann Hospital in Brighton, Massachusetts, and an assistant professor of medicine at Harvard Medical School. Dr. Siegel's interests in sports medicine dates back to 1976, when he ran his first marathon and began studies on medical complications of long-distance running. He has published numerous articles on muscle injury in marathon runners including evidence that long distance training alters the biochemical profile of the skeletal muscle to resemble a heart-muscle pattern. Skeletal muscle damage after marathon running creates elevations of cardiac enzymes in the blood resembling acute heart injury. Dr. Siegel works not only with runners but also with an eating disorders program at Hahnemann Hospital which is an outgrowth of his interest in exercise, body composition and health.*